Ketogenic Diet for Beginners

Your Guide for Success

Volume 3

L.B. Daniels

Printed in the United States of America

First Printing, 2017

Table of Contents

Chapter 1: Side Effects

Many diets have certain side effects or symptoms that you can look out for. Since you are manipulating your body into a state of ketosis, you are going to want to be extra sure that you pay attention to the potential side effects and symptoms. For many people, this is how they choose to monitor their keto levels and ensure that they are in a range that is successfully burning fat instead of sugar. For others, these symptoms may be scary when they are adjusting to their new diet, and they may wonder if what they are feeling is normal. In this chapter, we are going to thoroughly explore what you should expect to experience when you are on the keto diet. Understanding what is normal and what to look out for will help you feel more confident in your journey and what you are experiencing on the keto diet.

The Most Common Symptoms

There are many symptoms that people experience when they first take on the keto diet. These occur because your body is working to transition from gaining energy from carbohydrates to getting energy from fats. These symptoms rarely last too long, but can sometimes be difficult to endure. Once you get through them, however, you will feel a lot better and will start experiencing all of the benefits of keto.

Keto Flu

This is perhaps the most common symptom of the keto transition. It mimics flu-like symptoms because your body is getting used to the transition. You are likely to experience symptoms like nausea, headaches, a brain fog, and maybe even irritable. These symptoms generally disappear quickly, within' a few days once ketosis officially kicks in.

The main cause of the keto flu is generally dehydration, potentially combined with a salt deficiency. This happens when your urine production temporarily increases at the beginning of the keto journey, and can be easily cured with a few dietary additions. All you need to do is stay hydrated. The best way to do this when you are experiencing the keto flu is to add about a teaspoon of salt to your water and drink it. Alternatively, you can dissolve a bouillon cube into a cup of water and drink that. Doing this will help reduce or eliminate the symptoms of the keto flu within about half an hour. If you need to, you can do this once a day when you are in your first week, to help you cope with the keto flu symptoms. Make sure you don't abuse this cure, however, as adding excess salt to your diet can increase dehydration, and can also cause your blood pressures to rise excessively.

Another thing you need to make sure you're doing when you are experiencing the keto flu is to make sure that you are getting a lot of fat into your diet. Since you are no longer fueling your body with carbohydrates, you will need to make sure that you are getting enough fats to fuel your body. If you aren't, it may cause you to feel run down and extremely tired. You may also find that neither of these really help your symptoms go away. If that is the case, hang in there. They will usually go away within' a few days. If they persist for a long period of time, you should refrain from eating the keto way and discuss these symptoms with your doctor. He or she may be able to help you find out where you went wrong and address the situation.

Leg Cramps

When you are on a new diet such as the keto diet, you may find that you are getting frequent leg cramps. These are usually a minor issue, but they can sometimes be very painful. This is something that you experience due to your increased urine output decreasing the number of minerals in your body, specifically your magnesium levels. There are a few things that you can do to eliminate these symptoms. First, you want to make sure you are drinking plenty of water and that you are getting enough salt in your diet. So, the same thing you are doing for your keto flu (if you are using that strategy) should also assist you in eliminating these cramps. As well, you may choose to supplement yourself with some magnesium to help your body adjust.

Finally, if you really aren't finding any relief from the cramps and they are particularly painful, you may consider increasing your carb intake slightly, and then slowly weaning yourself off of them instead of going cold turkey. Leg cramps are a very common symptom and can generally be managed easily, you do not need to worry about this symptom becoming dangerous, as it won't.

Constipation

Due to your system needing to adjust to the changes in your diet, you may find that you are feeling constipated for some time when you first start your keto diet. This is completely normal, and there are a few things you can do to eliminate this symptom. First up, a lot of people don't drink nearly enough water, so increasing your fluid intake should also help you get things moving. As well, a lot of people don't ingest enough fiber during these early days of their keto diet, as they are not quite sure where they can get it from. Many people get their fiber from fruits, and don't realize that vegetables have a lot of fiber as well. You can get more fiber in your diet through eating raw vegetables to help get things moving.

Bad Breath

A common symptom of the keto diet is getting bad breath. This occurs because the acetone in your body increases, which can mean that the smell of your breath starts to remind people of nail polish remover. When your breath smells like this, it is a sign that your body is properly burning fat and making ketones. It may even be converting fat to ketones to fuel your brain. You may even discover that this smell comes out of you in the form of body odor, especially if you tend to work out and sweat a lot. While you aren't guaranteed to experience this symptom, it is a more common one. You can offset this one by drinking more fluid and getting enough salt, maintaining good oral hygiene practices, and using breath fresheners. Most often this symptom will go away within' a week or two, so you shouldn't wind up having it for a long period of time.

Heart Palpitations

Another symptom of dehydration and lack of salt in the diet that is common for people who just start the keto diet is heart palpitations. If you notice that your heart is beating slightly harder and faster than normal, it is nothing to worry about. The best way to make sure this doesn't happen, or to reduce it if it starts happening is to drink more water and slightly increase your salt intake. If you are on medications, suffer from any health symptoms or for any other reason should feel the need to be worried about your health, you should refrain from eating the keto diet and should talk to your doctor about this symptom. However, if you are not you should expect that this symptom will go away soon. The best thing you can do is make sure you are staying hydrated and that your salt intake stays up. It should not create any uncomfortable symptoms for you. Sometimes walking for a brisk 30 minutes each day will help your heart adjust to this diet as well.

Reduced Physical Performance

Adapting to this new energy form can sometimes take a few weeks. Because of this, you may notice that your physical performance is severely reduced for some time. This will not be a lasting change, and you should notice that it comes back after a short time. As with the other symptoms associated with the keto diet, you will need to increase your salt and water intake so that you stay hydrated. It should subside within' a few weeks, and then you will be back to your normal abilities. This is completely common and can be frustrating but it is not a long-term or lasting symptom.

Less Common Symptoms

There are some less common symptoms that go with the keto diet that you should look out for, as well. These symptoms are rarer to experience, but can still happen. It is a good idea to know what they are so that if you experience them you understand why, and what you can do about it. This will keep you from feeling as though you are really struggling to maintain the keto diet. Remember, these symptoms are less common so you are not as likely to get them. Still, you may experience them, so it's important to know what they are.

Temporary Hair Loss

When you have a major dietary change, especially one where you are transitioning from fueling your body with carbohydrates to fueling it with fat, you can end up with hormone fluctuations. This can cause you to start losing hair temporarily. This should not last long, and you should not lose much. It may seem alarming at first, but it will subside in no time. If you are going to experience this symptom, you won't start experiencing it right away. Instead, you will likely start experiencing it about 3-6 months into your diet. After a few months, it will stop and you won't even notice it anymore. The thinning that occurs will likely not be noticeable to others, just to yourself. If you increase your protein intake slightly, then this issue should not occur. Hair requires protein to be made and is mostly protein, so more protein would be a good idea.

Hair loss can also occur when you have been stressed out, so if you are feeling particularly stressed out, you will want to make sure that you are able to figure out why and learn to maintain your stress levels. This will increase your ability to regrow your hair and decrease the rate at which you are losing it. There isn't really anything else that you can do about this symptom, other than wait for it to go away. It shouldn't last too terribly long.

Elevated Cholesterol

Usually when you are on a low-carb high-fat diet, your cholesterol gets better. Sometimes, though, you will gain a slight elevation in your cholesterol when you start this diet. This elevation will generally actually be an increase in the *good* cholesterol, not the bad cholesterol. If it is an increase in the bad cholesterol, you will want to address the situation by understanding where you are getting your fat sources from. If you are eating too many saturated fats, or unhealthy fats, you will want to transition over to eating healthier fats. This will help decrease the amount of bad cholesterol in your system and make it easier for you to keep your levels healthy.

Reduced Alcohol Tolerance

Alcohol is largely produced by sugars, so when you are someone who does not ingest carbohydrates, you may find that you are a lot less tolerant to alcohol. You may find that you do not need as much to feel the effects. Because of this, you will need to be slow and careful about drinking alcohol to ensure that you aren't drinking more than your limit would be. In general, you don't want to ingest much alcohol when you are on the keto diet because it will take you out of ketosis. However, even a single cup may feel like a lot if you have been on keto for a long time. So, make sure that you are careful and slow about your intake so you don't accidentally overdo it. As well, make sure that you are not drinking it often, so that you don't break your ketosis and sabotage your diet.

Keto Rash

Some individuals who transition to the keto diet may develop a rash that sprawls across their chest and back. This is generally referred to as the "keto rash" and the exact cause is somewhat unknown. There are many theories as to why this happens, but no one is exactly sure. The typical conclusion is that it is caused by the ketones in the sweat. There are generally certain things that will worsen it, such as: entering ketosis and when the weather gets hot or they start sweating more.

These two things typically cause the rash to occur, and those who get it generally realize that the rash occurs where sweat would generally accumulate. It is assumed that this rash is caused by acetone exiting the body through sweat that then dries on the body. The best way to deal with this rash is to wear clothing that breathes, and change before your sweat dries. Also, shower regularly, especially after you've been exercising or sweating. If you struggle with the rash badly, you can exit ketosis by slightly increasing your carbohydrate intake to about 50-100 grams per day, and add intermittent fasting. Doing this will keep you on the low-carb diet and gaining some of the benefits, though you will not be gaining them as drastically. Still, if you are suffering with a rash it may be worthwhile. Finally, some people have used prescription ointments and antibiotics to help it, though this is not generally necessary.

Myths of Low Carb

A variety of myths have accumulated around the low-carb or keto diet that simply aren't true. These myths are often spread around the low-carb community, and it is important to realize that they are false. Those who spread these rumors are generally ones who are not fully educated on the diet, and who may not even be sure as to what it's total benefits are. Just to ensure that you are not falling victim to these myths, these are the ones that you are most likely to hear about:

Brain

Many people believe that your brain *needs* carbs to have enough energy to function properly. The truth is, when you are on the keto diet, your brain will be primarily fueled by fat, and it will still be healthy. The fat will get converted to ketones in your liver, which will turn into fuel for your brain. When this happens, your fat-burning will increase significantly, which is an awesome bonus for those looking to lose excess weight. As well, your body can produce glucose through a process that is called "gluconeogenesis" which means that it converts other nutrients to glucose to fuel your brain. You do not need to have carbohydrates in your diet to fuel your brain effectively and in a healthy way.

Ketoacidosis

There are many people who confuse ketosis with ketoacidosis and who believe that if you are on the keto diet you are at risk for entering a coma. The reality is that ketosis and ketoacidosis are *not* the same thing and when you are successfully on the keto diet, you are highly unlikely to enter ketoacidosis. The only ones who are highly at risk for ketoacidosis are those with diabetes type 1, which are typically not recommended to eat the keto diet in the first place. For the average healthy person, it can be very difficult to enter ketoacidosis. While it is a risk, it is not one that you need to be overly concerned about. If you are, you can speak with your doctor to formulate a clear list of symptoms that you should look out for, and what you should do if you start to experience them.

Gut Bacteria

While there are no conclusive studies done, a lot of research suggests that a low carb diet is *not* bad for your gut health. There is not a lot that can be said or confirmed about gut bacteria on the keto diet, so it is hard to report on this part. The best thing you can do to protect your gut health is to avoid using antibiotics unless you absolutely need them, and even then, you will want to make sure that you are not using as much. Make sure that when you are using them it is because it is mandatory, and not because it is a quick fix to something that could cure itself otherwise. To find out the exact answer for this, you can simply ask your doctor. "Are there any alternatives to antibiotics?" is a good question, as sometimes your doctor may have an alternative. Other times, they may not. While you should never defy your doctor's judgment, you are always welcome to ask questions when you are unsure about something.

Deficiencies

Many people believe that because you are cutting out a major food group with the keto diet that you are going to end up with deficiencies. This can be even further assumed from those who read the symptoms and see that many symptoms can arise in the first few weeks due to decreased salt intake, or a salt deficiency. The reality is that when you are on the keto diet and you learn to maintain it properly, you are not going to be deficient in anything. In fact, the simple fact that you are not able to rely on carbohydrates to fill you up will often mean that you are eating an even more well-rounded diet than you were before, meaning that you are going to be less likely to be deficient, not more likely to be

Taking one multi-vitamin each day will cover everything. Like it was stated before, major vitamins such as A D E and K require adequate fat intake to be absorbed properly, so a person on a low fat diet may actually be worse off than someone on a ketogenic diet.

Thyroid

If you are eating a well-formulated low-carb diet that is nutrient rich and healthy for you, you are not likely to experience anything wrong with your thyroid. Long-term starvation or calorie restrictions can lead to hypothyroidism, but since this diet does not contain any restrictions or starvation, you should be fine. As a matter of fact, many individuals who transition to the keto diet find that their preexisting thyroid issues reverse or become cured because of their new dietary style. Again, you will never want to stop taking medications or change your treatments on your own. Always make sure that you are working closely with your doctor to monitor these concerns and ensure that you are not at risk for producing damage.

Kidneys

It is highly unlikely that eating a low-carb diet will affect your kidneys in any negative way. A well-formulated low-carb diet should be high in fat, not protein, which is what will make this a healthy diet. If you are eating too much protein, *then* you may experience issues as a result. However, it is unlikely that you will experience any of these issues with your kidney if you are eating healthily. For those who have healthy functioning kidneys, there should be no issue eating a low-carb diet.

However, if you have a severely damaged kidney or kidneys, you will want to discuss the keto diet with your doctor, as you will have special dietary conditions you should follow to maintain your kidney health.

Depression

When you are on the low-carb diet, you may experience symptoms that are like depression for the first week or two while your body adjusts. These symptoms might include lethargy, excess fatigue, irritability, brain fog, and more. However, this will subside within' a week or two and then you will be back to your normal condition. This usually occurs when you are not getting enough fluids and salts. Long term, you will be more likely to find the opposite to be true. The keto diet is excellent for helping people reduce symptoms of depression and feel healthier overall.

Osteoporosis

Many places have spread rumors that if you are eating a low-carb diet, then you are at risk for your "acidic" blood leaching minerals from your bones. As a result, they believe that a low-carb diet can lead to conditions like osteoporosis. This is actually false, and the myth has been debunked by several credible sources. Under normal circumstances, when you are on a keto diet your blood pH levels don't change, depending on what you are eating. The blood pH is controlled within' a very narrow span based on your body's natural and healthy functions, because if it weren't you would die. You do not have to worry about what a ketogenic diet may do to your bones, because the reality is that it will do nothing. At most, it will make them healthier, not weaker.

There are several potential side effects that you may experience as a result of being on a keto diet. For the most part, these side effects are unlikely and if you do experience them, they won't last a long period of time. A couple of weeks, at most. These symptoms are generally the result of temporary increased urine output which can cause temporary dehydration, as well as your body not having enough salt in it. For most these symptoms, you can control and eliminate them by simply drinking more water and including a little extra salt in your diet.

If your symptoms are extremely insufferable and you are struggling with them badly, you may consider adding a few extra grams of carbs in your diet and then slowly eliminating them as you work into a deeper state of ketosis. Or, you may simply desire to maintain a lessened state of ketosis, where you will still get the benefits to a degree. However, if your symptoms become terrible and you are extremely affected by them, you will want to make sure that you are talking to your doctor and that you stop eating the keto diet. There may be an underlying condition that does not respond well to a low-carb diet.

Chapter 2: Tips and Tricks

There are a few ways that you can make the keto diet even easier for you to maintain. These tips and tricks will give you the opportunity to really make your keto diet effective and easy to achieve.

Meal Prep

A great way to stay on track with your keto diet is to meal prep. Meal prepping allows you to pre-make your keto friendly meals in advance, and all you will have to do is heat them up when you are ready to eat them. Most meal preps can be created a few days in advance, so you can pre-make them before you're going to need them, and simply eat your meal preps for a few days. It is not abnormal to prepare your meals for a week at a time as many athletes swear by this method.

Journal Your Intake

Journaling what you have been eating is a great option when you are on the keto diet. It lets you know exactly how many carbs you have been eating, as well as how much protein and fat you have been eating. You can monitor what recipes you liked and didn't like, what foods made you feel certain ways, and what types of things trigger you to crave carbohydrates. This can make the transition significantly smoother, and it is even suggested for you to maintain your keto diary or journal well into your experience, to ensure that you are staying on top of what you are eating and how your experience has been so far.

You may even want to track your measurements to see how your weight loss journey has been going, and what methods you used that helped you eliminate weight quickly and easily!

Learn to Monitor Through Symptoms

It is handy having a blood monitor or urine test strips to check your state of ketosis. However, it can become tiresome having to check this constantly to see if you are in a state of ketosis. At first, these are extremely handy. Over time, though, you should consider learning how you can monitor your ketosis through symptoms. This is where a journal comes in handy, too. Being able to monitor your ketosis through symptoms means that you will not have to test constantly to ensure that you are in ketosis. Instead, you will know you are and you will know what you need to do to maintain it.

Have "Cheat Days"

As you may have noticed in the "what to eat" section, there are some foods you can eat occasionally, such as a slice or two of bread, a couple of berries, a glass of alcohol, or a slice of dark chocolate. It can be helpful to have specific cheat days in your schedule where you will allow yourself to eat these items in moderate amounts. Having pre-chosen cheat days is a great way to make sure that you can indulge in the foods you like, without feeling like you want to eat them every day. If you don't have pre-set cheat days, there is a chance that you could end up having cheat days more often than normal, which could sabotage your diet.

Alternatively, you may starve yourself of your cheat foods and eventually have a major crash and destroy your ketosis altogether, because you couldn't say no any longer. It is very handy to have cheat days!

Join a Support Society

There are many online societies on the internet for you to join that will help you maintain your keto diet. These societies are great because the people in them are at all different stages of their diet, so some may directly relate to what you are experiencing, and others will remember what it is like and have tips or words of motivation to keep you going. These support societies are especially good if you are the only one in your family switching to a low-carb diet, as it will make it easier for you to speak to people who understand you when your family may not understand what you are going through. Check google for any type of forum you can join!

Prepare for Symptoms and Side Effects
A good idea when you are transitioning into a keto diet is to ensure that you are prepared for the symptoms and side effects that you are bound to experience. Even if you don't experience them all, you are going to end up experiencing some of them. Having yourself mentally prepared for these side effects, as well as understanding what you can do to make them better will help you when you are starting out on your keto journey and are facing them along the way.

Keep a Cheat Sheet

It can be very handy to keep a cheat sheet in your purse or wallet when you are leaving the house, especially if you plan on eating out. You can even have one in your kitchen. Doing this will help you remember what is keto friendly and what isn't. It will make ordering and making food much easier, because you won't have to play the guessing game or spend time researching it.

Chapter 3: Success at the Ketogenic Diet

The keto diet is a low-carb high-fat diet that is excellent for many different reasons. If you are seeking to lose weight, manage your risk of contracting diseases, or manage symptoms of ailments you already live with, the keto diet can offer you some serious help. While there are some people who should not eat the keto diet, the majority of individuals can eat this way.

At first, the keto diet may seem difficult to eat, as it can be hard to cut out all your favorite foods. In our society, fruits, pastas, breads, treats and other carbohydrate-rich foods are staples. It can be hard to remove these favorites and feel as though you are depriving yourself from them. However, once you grow accustomed to the keto diet, you will find that it is a lot easier for you to maintain, and that soon you won't crave these foods at all. In fact, you might even stop liking them altogether.

The keto diet has many health benefits, and is often recommended by doctors for all the wonders it can work on the human body. Some of the awesome outcomes you are likely to experience from the keto diet include:

- Freedom from sugar cravings, food fixations and hypoglycemia
- Freedom from excessive hunger
- Reduced blood pressure levels
- Drop in bad cholesterols
- A drop in your triglyceride levels
- Drop in blood sugar and insulin levels
- Increased energy levels
- Decreased joint pains and stiffness
- Eliminate brain fog and increase mental clarity
- Improved sleep patterns and decreased sleep apnea symptoms
- Effortless weight loss
- Relief from heartburn symptoms
- Reduced instance of gum disease and tooth decay
- Increased healthier digestion and gut health
- Better moods overall

There are many reasons why this diet is recommended for individuals. Those with type 2 diabetes, thyroid issues, epilepsy, and other health ailments are often recommended to eat this way by their doctor. Others prefer to eat this way because it can help with losing weight. Even many body builders and high-performance athletes like to eat this diet because it helps them build muscle mass and prevent the buildup of excess fats. There are a few variations of this diet, three of which are more advanced versions that are often consumed by those who are body builders or high-performance athletes. The average person, however, will simply eat the Standard Keto Diet to get all the best benefits from it.

The keto diet has many myths around it, most of which come from inconclusive results that are driven from fear-based pseudoscience. Virtually these myths can be debunked or figured out when you consider them. Some of these myths arise from individuals who take information based around specialized variation of the keto diet and spread it around as though it were to apply to all people. For example, the idea that ketosis and ketoacidosis are the same thing. This is a major myth that is simply not true.

The keto diet is one that can take a few weeks to become used to. There are many symptoms you may experience as you switch from fueling your body with carbohydrates, over to fueling your body with fats. This can cause you to feel symptoms such as the keto flu, leg cramping, and more. These are generally temporary, and can be easily managed with some slight adjustments to your water and salt intake.

This book is the perfect guide to walk you through all the steps of eating the keto way. You will learn to understand what the keto diet is, how to get into and maintain ketosis, what it means to eat a keto diet, and easy steps for maintaining it. You will also learn about common symptoms and side effects and how you can easily manage them in your life. This guidebook is a great pocket-guide to keep on hand when you are transitioning to a keto diet. It will help you ensure that you are doing it properly and safely, and that you are gaining the maximum benefit from your new diet change.

Each section and chapter was written for your maximum reader enjoyment. It is my sincere hope that you can gain plenty of information from this book, and that you are able to use it to help you effortlessly transition to the keto diet Please take your time, and enjoy it. Feel free to keep it on hand so that you can easily refer to it along your path, and ensure that you are eating the keto way, the right way.

Journaling for Success

There are many things that you can do to make your keto diet easier, and you will learn about more along the way. Most of the tips and tricks you start to live by will be ones that you create yourself as you gain experience in the diet the longer you go along. Therefore, it is particularly helpful to keep a journal, as you can jot these notes down and create your own guide to go by as you are on your keto journey.

Chapter 4: Is Exercise Necessary?

As stated in volume 1 and 2, exercise and working out is important, but not nearly as important as the food you eat, what type of food you eat, but most importantly, the calories in those foods you eat, that regulate your body mass. If you force your body to burn calories then when you are at rest you may burn less calories to a certain degree. Athletes have such low heart rates when at rest because when they burn many calories during the day they have ended up training their body to burn less calories when they aren't exercising. The human body has a way of balancing itself out. If you are cold, your body heat turns up, if you are hot, you sweat to cool down. If you force your body to burn calories, you will train your body to burn calories less in other ways.

One way an individual may believe exercise burns calories is that just having an exercise routine causes a person to clean up their food intake. Also, individuals that tend to exercise a lot typically use a supplement that contains caffeine (even if it is just coffee), which suppresses appetite and causes you to fidget more and move more altogether. Even if the body tries to regulate how many calories it wants to burn, if you exercise a lot, you will burn more calories than your body can down regulate during the other parts of the day.

One way for your body to down-regulate its caloric burning properties if you do a lot of cardiovascular activities is to burn off some muscle, so you look less lean and more like a marathon runner. Have you ever seen a marathon runner? They are very slim and frail looking because they have burned off a lot of their muscles from all the cardiovascular exercise they are doing to prepare for their marathons. Look at a sprinter, they train with sprints for their cardio, and they also take on resistance training for their bursts of speed. Marathon runners don't generally do resistance training as they need to be as light as possible.

Exercise is great, but it is something you add on to a healthy eating plan to maximize your weight loss. If you were to compare the two types of exercise, cardiovascular exercise (cardio), or resistance training (lifting weight and the such), you may want to look to resistance training, as you build muscle and tone your body in addition to burning calories. Cardio just aims to burn calories and your body will build a tolerance to that, but the tolerance your body creates to resistance training is strength, more muscle and tone, which burns more calories when at rest than cardio.

Exercise is good for health, but don't do too much. Moderation is the key, and this goes with cardio and resistance training and eating healthy. You need to create a balance. Weight gain is mostly from two things: Too many calories from foods you eat during the day followed by too much inactivity. Some individuals may thing their lack of activity is what caused their weight gain, but it's not so true in the way that they think. It isn't because you are burning less calories during the day, it is because inactivity causes boredom and boredom causes you to want to eat more. We will go through this in further chapters.

Chapter 5: Burning Calories

As said in volume 1 and 2, calories are the form of energy we get out of food. If you take a "calorimeter", which is a certain heating device, and toss various foods in it, you get a certain number of calories burnt out of it. Toss in some steak, calories. Toss in some bread, calories. Toss in some broccoli, calories. Toss in the insides of a tree, you get calories. For the tree, yes, in Papua New Guinea they eat the inside of trees, and they have generally the same caloric value as potatoes. Hell, let's go ahead and toss in Gasoline into that calorimeter (Don't drink gasoline, please!), and you get calories. Okay, so gasoline makes a car run, right? Well it's the calories that do it. It's the heat that is generated that does it. For example, a calorie is the energy needed to increase the temperature of a given mass of water by 1 degrees Celsius.

Let's view the human body as a machine for a second. It takes a lot of food each day to run, and specific foods give off certain kinds of macronutrients and micronutrients, sure. But in the end of all things, what makes the human body run is Calories. The average man, regardless of bodyweight to an extent, needs about 2700 calories a day to stay the same weight. If this man is 150 pounds, or 300 pounds, about 2700 calories will keep him that weight. A woman needs about 2100 calories per day to maintain any weight she is at as well under the same circumstances.

Exercise increases how many calories you burn, in which makes you lose weight, but as stated in previous chapters, your body will fight back to balance out your expenditure. Your body has one job, and one job only: to keep you alive. If you stress it, it will find a way to cope with that stress and you become stronger. If a marathon runner runs many hours a day, the body will view that as stress and make it easier to run for hours a day, be it a lower heart rate, less muscle mass, and of course less body fat.

Calories are the units of energy your body uses to maintain your body through all bodily processes during the day. That is over-simplifying it because when you say a man burns about 2700 calories a day and a woman burns about 2100 calories a day, this is taking in all different processes that are going on under the hood, so to speak.

For the three macro-nutrients: Protein, Carbohydrates, and Fat, they all have various modes of action. When your body burns them, they give off a certain caloric value: Protein and Carbohydrates burn at about 4 calories for each gram, and fat burns at about 9 calories per gram. It may look simple to remove fat from your diet to lose weight, but luckily it makes you feel fuller than carbohydrates and protein to a certain degree.

Carbohydrates are burned and turned into glucose to keep your blood sugar (energy) regulated. Your body can only have about one teaspoon of glucose in your bloodstream at one time or you will die, so your body uses the hormones insulin and glucagon to keep it going and coming. Protein and Dietary fat is used for various hormone production. Protein can turn into glucose when burned as well, but the body does not prefer it, and dietary fat can be used as energy as ketones when your blood sugar is low as well.

Chapter 6: Reducing Body Fat

Just like volume 1 and 2 implies, for basic measures, a pound of fat when burned by the human body, is about 3500 calories. If a man (burning 2700 calories a day), eats about 2200 calories, he will have burned about 500 more than he ate, which in turn the body required from his body fat, so he would be at a "deficit" for the day of about -500. If this man did this for 7 days straight, he would be at a deficit of about 3500 calories, and in return, he would have burned about 1 pound of fat from his body in various locations. That's all. For the same thing to happen for a woman that burns about 2100 calories a day, a woman would just need to eat 1600 calories. Women burn about 2100 calories per day because of less muscle mass, but luckily, they have less of an appetite to compensate so to speak.

If a person, regardless of their current bodyweight, eats roughly 500 calories more than they burn each day, and does this for about 7 days, they will gain one pound of fat somewhere on their body in various locations. Do this for 52 weeks or one year, and there is your 50+ pound weight gain that just snuck up on you. This is exactly how body weight loss and gain happens. You put food in, and calories come out.

For general information, according to volume 1 and 2, the hormone that tells you to stop eating is called leptin. The other hormone that tells you to eat is ghrelin. If you eat foods with high sugar content, your blood sugar will spike, and your pancreas will release a hormone called insulin, and this will drive your blood sugar back down. But, this also means you will have lower blood sugar now, so you will feel weak and low on energy and hungry again, so your body will release ghrelin to get you to eat again.

Ever eat Chinese food? Have you ever felt hungry again an hour or so later? This is exactly that, but it also works with high sugar or high carbohydrate foods. Therefore, a lower carbohydrate diet may be good for you, but it doesn't mean it's the best solution, it just means watch out for foods that spike your blood sugar too high, like rice, pasta, potatoes, sugar, candy and sodas.

What this all means is that individuals may have trouble with their appetites, and their body's mechanisms will make them eat depending on the foods they eat, but when it comes down to it, it still matters about calories. Yes, certain eating patterns and selections of food have certain amounts of calories, but these calories may be adjusting your leptin and ghrelin signals to make you eat irregularly. If you ignored these signals and ate a specific number of calories each day to lose weight, you would succeed.

A lot of diets try to get around this and tell you to eat certain types of foods in hopes that this signaling puts you in a caloric deficit without getting too complex about things. It works for some people, and it doesn't work for some people. It honestly really depends. If you don't like to eat too much and go on an Atkins style diet, you may lose weight because not only does protein and dietary fat cause your appetite to be suppressed, you don't like eating that way anyway. But losing weight isn't about dieting and getting off diets back and forth, that can't be healthy mentally and physically.

So, if you are put on an Atkins style diet, lose some weight, and return to your normal eating, you will gain the weight back because you did not make any lasting changes. A lasting change to something like that would be to incorporate meat into your normal food schedules if you didn't eat that much meat before, so that may help with suppressing your appetite.

There are individuals that have lost weight on a 'Twinkie' style diet, by just eating about 1800 calories a day and proceed about two pounds of fat loss each week until they decided to return to normal eating. That is interesting, because eating only addicting foods can be a challenge, but they did it. Eating only junk food though also means you will not be getting any vitamins or minerals to keep you healthy, so I hope those individuals also took a multi vitamin at the very least.

Chapter 8: Food Journals

Just like in volume 1 and 2, sometimes, losing weight could be as simple as looking at what you are eating. It is very easy to just wake up, eat whatever you see in the kitchen or whatever is nearby or looks good on the way to work. It's easy to grab a snack or two at work and drop by a fast food restaurant on the way home after it all. Sometimes foods don't look so fattening or high in calories, so it is easy to live each day thinking everything is okay, when the weight is creeping up.

What this means is, if you do anything to start any program, to ease into it, you may want to take a week or two and just write down everything you are eating. Just this might take care of things. There is such a thing in psychology of cash versus credit cards, it is much easier to swipe your credit card and forget you bought that item versus handing out actual cash, your brain registers it differently, so with that said, mindlessly eating food versus just writing it down may reduce your food consumption to the point that your weight reduces enough to make you happy to start.

If after a week or two things are not taking care of themselves, then look at how you are recording your food consumption. Writing "a slice of pizza" is different than saying you had "a large slice of meat lover's pizza" from your favorite restaurant that loves to top off your pizzas with ingredients. For general knowledge, if you only drink diet soda, they are useful because they have no calories, but the artificial sweeteners can increase appetite, so be weary.

Chapter 9: Weigh Once Per Week

Volume 1 and 2 states that a lot of individuals take on a weight loss journey, but weigh themselves many times a day or at times that are not consistent. It is very easy to weight yourself in the morning and by the time you go to sleep to weight yourself and wonder where many pounds came from. Of course, food has weight, but how does this change from the time you fall asleep and wake up? Water. As you sleep, your body will expel water at a very slow rate as well as when you wake up you will typically use the restroom, so that extra weight goes away.

Some individuals also choose to weigh each day, or every couple day, being very inconsistent, which makes one bad day make someone think that their weight loss efforts are not working. For example, even if you did not eat too much, if you ate fast food or take out one night, that type of food may be high in carbohydrates and very high in sodium, which binds to water that you ingest for a few days, so the next day you may appear to have gained body fat, when it was just water.

From here, just take note to weigh yourself once a week under the same conditions. For example, I like to weigh myself on Saturday morning as soon as I wake up, right after using the restroom and brushing my teeth. I do this for 4 weeks and take note to my weight as it changes. If my weight stays the same each week or increases, then I know I need to pull back my food intake and/or calories.

Chapter 10: Why Do Diets Fail Sometimes?

Let's be honest, as stated in volume 2, are you just tired of all these diets out there? There seems to be a diet created by everyone that is supposed to work. What about all these diets that claim that their diet is the only one that works? How about the diets that claim amazing health benefits but don't help with weight loss? Or how about the ones that help with weight loss but don't help with health benefits? You have diets that want you drinking special teas and you have diets that want you to drink weight loss shakes. You also have diets that want you to eat only vegetables, you have diets that want you to eat only meat, you have diets that say that you should stay away from breads and pastas, and the list goes on. When will this all stop? Eat the way you want to, life is short. Balancing health and the proper about of calories you eat day will lead to a slim, healthy you, you do not need to go to the extremes for these things.

There's only a specific amount of foods in the world, and taking one of two food groups away might help you in the short term or even in the long run, but do any of these diets tell you why this works? Sure, they might tell you why, but do they tell you *why?* This is what I'm asking you, because a lot of diets will speak about their health benefits but not tell you much about what's not so good about the diet.

What if I told you that eating any way you want in terms of foods, can give you the weight loss you desire. No, this isn't some one simple trick or one amazing secret type of book, but it could be. Let me explain: Calories.

The reason diets work is they somehow get you to eat less calories which result in weight loss. Some individuals like these diets so much that the diet fails to reduce their food consumption, so they gain weight eventually. The famous "Atkins" type style diet wants you eating meat to reduce your appetite, but if you love meat, you'll gain weight soon.

Do you know anyone that went on a health kick? They drank only juice for a week or two to 'detox' and to lose some weight. Why did this work or fail? For one thing, drinking only juices all day may lead to a significant number of caloric deficits, and in return will make the person lose weight. Also, because juice has barely any bulk weight, you will lose the general weight that your body retains from a normal digestion system.

So, your friend returns to eating normally after eating some things that they crave because they were restricting themselves, and now they gained their bulk weight back and may have gained some weight from their cravings. But at least they were detoxing for a week, right?

Some individuals can drink so much juice on their juice fast that they don't lose any body fat and just some bulk weight. All that work and they didn't even get to eat solid foods the entire time. Sure, if you like that, do it, but if you do it for some magically benefits, don't do it. Balance is the key, you can drink juice and such during the day and have some nice solid foods at night, you don't have to go into the extremes for a week for significant results, because they will go away when the health kick is over.

Chapter 11: Junk Food

As stated in volume 2, Let's look at "junk food". Why is this called junk food in the first place? Well because it doesn't supply you with any good micro nutrients (vitamins and minerals). Also, junk food is usually very high in calories (We can use the term calorie-dense). Twinkies are tasty, but they have barely any vitamins, minerals, and they have a lot of calories, and tend to increase your appetite as well. The junk food and fast food industry know that combining dietary fat, unhealthy carbohydrates, and salt can produce an addiction in the human brain, so they use that to their advantage to sell more and more products.

Ever wonder why you can eat a bag of potato chips and it feels like you didn't eat anything, but you are still hungry and want more? How come it is difficult to eat only one or two slices of pizza or just one cheeseburger and a small order of fries? The specific combination of macro nutrients produces that addiction effect and you want more, and on top of all of that, it messes with your blood sugar, causing it to go up very high and then crashing, making you also want to eat more as well.

Junk food is coined junk food also because it is so calorie-dense, that for how many calories you eat, you barely get any 'bulk'. There are about two ways for your body to signal to your brain that you have eaten and are done. The first way is at the bottom of your stomach, when you eat food, your stomach lining stretches and then that signals to your brain that you have eaten, and then your brain signals to your body to stop eating for now or you will feel uncomfortable.

Another way for your body to signal that you have eaten is once food is in the bottom of your stomach, it empties into your small intestine as liquid chyme, and all the nutrients start to go down your intestines, which then signals to your brain that you have eaten as well. Have you ever seen someone pile food into their stomach and seem like they can keep going and going? That is because they may have a faulty stomach processing switch and must rely on their small intestines to send the signal instead.

What this all means is that when you eat 'junk food' you end up filling the bottom of your stomach much less than if it was a healthier version of food, and there for you end up eating more calories. This is exactly why it's a good idea to stay away from chips, sodas, and candy and lean towards green vegetables without adding any special sauces to them to increase the flavor. Sure, you can add melted cheese to steamed broccoli, but now you are making it have the calories of a junk food with some health benefits. Sometimes just removing added sauces and such from prepared foods is enough to cause an individual to lose weight.

Fast food tends to be very packed with calories from the macronutrient fat, and somewhat from carbohydrates. Would it surprise you to know that fast food restaurants ad a small amount of sugar to their hamburger buns to increase their desirability? Interesting stuff. There was a documentary in past years that a man ate only McDonalds three times a day for a month and gained about twenty pounds. This makes McDonalds look bad, right? Not so close, many individuals get away with eating fast-food, but they count their calories. The only problem here is they are succeeding at an uphill battle because fast food is addicting.

Chapter 12: Losing Weight and Keeping It Off

As said in previous chapters, the human body burns calories. The average male burns 2700 calories each day, and the average woman burns 2100 calories each day. If you eat 500 calories a day less than you burn, and do this for 7 days, you will burn one pound of body fat. This is called the Law of Conservation of Energy. You may lose more than a pound a week this way as your body will also release stored toxins and water, so if you do this for one month, not only will you lose about four pounds, but you may lose another 5 to 10 pounds from just stored toxins, your body usually only releases this when you lose body fat.

If you started to over-eat again and began gaining weight, your body will build up toxins and water again and you'll gain that excess weight back. This is the coined 'Yo-Yo dieting" issue. Don't worry about it too much, but it is a nice bonus when you start losing weight, and it isn't so great if you start gaining weight again, but the point is to not gain weight anymore, so that will be just fine.

For men: Eat 2200 calories a day. For Women, eat 1600 calories a day. Read the nutrition labels properly and measure your calories, and if what you are eating does not have a nutrition label, type it into google and you will find many websites that have calculated that for you. Do not pick the item with the lowest number, pick the median one as you don't want to cheat yourself and confuse yourself as you just miscalculated your caloric totals.

Bonus 1: Weight Loss Template

As stated in volume 1 and 2, journaling your food intake is a must when it comes to weight loss. One of the major reasons weight gain slowly creeps up on an individual is that they are not paying attention to what they are eating and accidently overconsume enough to cause weight gain. It is very easy to mindlessly consume food when you have a busy, hectic and on the go schedule, but that makes weight gain easy. It is time to start journaling your food intake.

If you purchased the paperback version of this book, below is a 2-week weight loss template that you should fill out each day. As you fill out the template with what you ate and drank each day, on day 7 and 14, weigh yourself and record your bodyweight. This will tell you if you are making any progress with your eating plan. You can weigh yourself more frequently, but it is advised to do it every seven days for more accurate results.

After you complete the fourteen-day weight loss template, I have also created an advanced weight loss template that will help you understand your weight loss and/or weight stall if you still are stalling. Keep it up and you will find losing weight is simple and fun! Patience is the best variable when it comes to weight loss.

Weight Loss Template

Day 1   **Weight** ______

Directions:

Write your food and drink intake as accurately as you can. Each day you will get better at doing so.

____
____
____
____
____
____
____
____
____
____
____
____
____
____
____
____
____
____
____
____

Weight Loss Template

Day 2

Directions:

Write your food and drink intake as accurately as you can. Each day you will get better at doing so.

Weight Loss Template

Day 3

Directions:

Write your food and drink intake as accurately as you can. Each day you will get better at doing so.

Weight Loss Template

Day 4

Directions:

Write your food and drink intake as accurately as you can. Each day you will get better at doing so.

Weight Loss Template

Day 5

Directions:

Write your food and drink intake as accurately as you can. Each day you will get better at doing so.

Weight Loss Template

Day 6

Directions:

Write your food and drink intake as accurately as you can. Each day you will get better at doing so.

____

____

____

____

____

____

____

____

____

____

____

____

____

____

____

____

____

____

____

____

____

____

Weight Loss Template

Day 7   **Weight** _______

Directions:

Write your food and drink intake as accurately as you can. Each day you will get better at doing so.

____

____

____

____

____

____

____

____

____

____

____

____

____

____

____

____

____

____

____

____

Weight Loss Template

Day 8

Directions:

Write your food and drink intake as accurately as you can. Each day you will get better at doing so.

Weight Loss Template

Day 9

Directions:

Write your food and drink intake as accurately as you can. Each day you will get better at doing so.

Weight Loss Template

Day 10

Directions:

Write your food and drink intake as accurately as you can. Each day you will get better at doing so.

Weight Loss Template

Day 11

Directions:

Write your food and drink intake as accurately as you can. Each day you will get better at doing so.

Weight Loss Template

Day 12

Directions:

Write your food and drink intake as accurately as you can. Each day you will get better at doing so.

Weight Loss Template

Day 13

Directions:

Write your food and drink intake as accurately as you can. Each day you will get better at doing so.

Weight Loss Template

Day 14   **Weight** ______

Directions:

Write your food and drink intake as accurately as you can. Each day you will get better at doing so.

Bonus 2: Advanced Weight Loss Template

Congratulations on reaching day 14 on the weight loss template for volume 2 and hopefully volume 1 and 2! How was journaling your food intake? Did your weight change? Let's go into some details about weight loss that will help you in further progress or help you get over a hurdle. Weight loss is simple, but it also can be complicated if you let it be.

As stated in volume 1, all food is made up of three macronutrients: Protein, Carbohydrates, and Dietary Fat. Protein and Carbohydrates have a caloric value of 4 calories per gram, and dietary fat has a caloric value of 9 calories per gram.

What is a calorie you say? It is the type of energy your body extracts out of the food you eat. The average man needs 2700 calories each day to maintain his weight, and the average woman requires 2100 calories per day.

A pound of fat on the human body has a value of 3500 calories. For example, as a woman, if you ate 1600 calories each day, you would technically be in a deficit of 500 calories for that day. If you did this for one week, you would lose exactly one pound of fat and additionally, your body would purge some toxins from your body fat as well.

In addition to journaling your food intake, please record the calories in these foods you are eating. If there are no nutrition facts label on the products you are eating, do a google search on what you ate and there should be a website that has calculated it for you.

Advanced Weight Loss Template

Day 1   Weight ______

Directions:

Write your food and drink intake as accurately as you can. Write the calories to the right.

______________________________________   ______

______________________________________   ______

______________________________________   ______

______________________________________   ______

______________________________________   ______

______________________________________   ______

______________________________________   ______

______________________________________   ______

______________________________________   ______

______________________________________   ______

______________________________________   ______

______________________________________   ______

______________________________________   ______

Total   ______

Advanced Weight Loss Template

Day 2

Directions:

Write your food and drink intake as accurately as you can. Write the calories to the right.

Total _____

Advanced Weight Loss Template

Day 3

Directions:

Write your food and drink intake as accurately as you can. Write the calories to the right.

__________________________________ ______

__________________________________ ______

__________________________________ ______

__________________________________ ______

__________________________________ ______

__________________________________ ______

__________________________________ ______

__________________________________ ______

__________________________________ ______

__________________________________ ______

__________________________________ ______

__________________________________ ______

Total ______

Advanced Weight Loss Template

Day 4

Directions:

Write your food and drink intake as accurately as you can. Write the calories to the right.

____   ______

____   ______

____   ______

____   ______

____   ______

____   ______

____   ______

____   ______

____   ______

____   ______

____   ______

____   ______

Total   ______

Advanced Weight Loss Template

Day 5

Directions:

Write your food and drink intake as accurately as you can. Write the calories to the right.

_______________________________________ _______

_______________________________________ _______

_______________________________________ _______

_______________________________________ _______

_______________________________________ _______

_______________________________________ _______

_______________________________________ _______

_______________________________________ _______

_______________________________________ _______

_______________________________________ _______

_______________________________________ _______

_______________________________________ _______

_______________________________________ _______

Total _______

Advanced Weight Loss Template

Day 6

Directions:

Write your food and drink intake as accurately as you can. Write the calories to the right.

____________________________________ ______

____________________________________ ______

____________________________________ ______

____________________________________ ______

____________________________________ ______

____________________________________ ______

____________________________________ ______

____________________________________ ______

____________________________________ ______

____________________________________ ______

____________________________________ ______

____________________________________ ______

Total ______

Advanced Weight Loss Template

Day 7   Weight ______

Directions:

Write your food and drink intake as accurately as you can. Write the calories to the right.

____   ______

____   ______

____   ______

____   ______

____   ______

____   ______

____   ______

____   ______

____   ______

____   ______

____   ______

____   ______

____   ______

Total   ______

Advanced Weight Loss Template

Day 8

Directions:

Write your food and drink intake as accurately as you can. Write the calories to the right.

_____________________________________   _______

_____________________________________   _______

_____________________________________   _______

_____________________________________   _______

_____________________________________   _______

_____________________________________   _______

_____________________________________   _______

_____________________________________   _______

_____________________________________   _______

_____________________________________   _______

_____________________________________   _______

_____________________________________   _______

_____________________________________   _______

Total   _______

Advanced Weight Loss Template

Day 9

Directions:

Write your food and drink intake as accurately as you can. Write the calories to the right.

____   ______

____   ______

____   ______

____   ______

____   ______

____   ______

____   ______

____   ______

____   ______

____   ______

____   ______

____   ______

____   ______

Total   ______

Advanced Weight Loss Template

Day 10

Directions:

Write your food and drink intake as accurately as you can. Write the calories to the right.

Total _____

Advanced Weight Loss Template

Day 11

Directions:

Write your food and drink intake as accurately as you can. Write the calories to the right.

_____________________________________   _____

_____________________________________   _____

_____________________________________   _____

_____________________________________   _____

_____________________________________   _____

_____________________________________   _____

_____________________________________   _____

_____________________________________   _____

_____________________________________   _____

_____________________________________   _____

_____________________________________   _____

_____________________________________   _____

_____________________________________   _____

Total   ______

Advanced Weight Loss Template

Day 12

Directions:

Write your food and drink intake as accurately as you can. Write the calories to the right.

____   _______

____   _______

____   _______

____   _______

____   _______

____   _______

____   _______

____   _______

____   _______

____   _______

____   _______

____   _______

____   _______

Total   _______

Advanced Weight Loss Template

Day 13

Directions:

Write your food and drink intake as accurately as you can. Write the calories to the right.

________________________________ _____

________________________________ _____

________________________________ _____

________________________________ _____

________________________________ _____

________________________________ _____

________________________________ _____

________________________________ _____

________________________________ _____

________________________________ _____

________________________________ _____

________________________________ _____

Total _____

Advanced Weight Loss Template

Day 14   Weight _______

Directions:

Write your food and drink intake as accurately as you can. Write the calories to the right.

_______________________________________   _______

_______________________________________   _______

_______________________________________   _______

_______________________________________   _______

_______________________________________   _______

_______________________________________   _______

_______________________________________   _______

_______________________________________   _______

_______________________________________   _______

_______________________________________   _______

_______________________________________   _______

_______________________________________   _______

_______________________________________   _______

                                    Total _______

Conclusion

As stated in volume 1 and 2, weight loss is a life-long journey, but it does not have to be painful. Individuals are so busy with their lives that they end up eating on the go, and just enjoying life a little too much, but this in turn creates a problem, a weight problem. Think of it this way, if you went to purchase something, how would you feel if you swiped a credit card, grabbed the receipt, tossed it into the trash and went on with your business? Compare to that to seeing the price tag of the items you bought and had to physically give cash for the items you purchased. After that, receive the receipt and look at what you purchased? Which scenario would help you regulate your costs and reduce the chance you would go into debt?

This applies to weight loss the same way but in reverse, instead of going into debt, you gain weight. It's that simple, but also complex if you are used to eating anything when you have the time or when you have a craving and such.

I hope you enjoyed this book and hope you become successful in your weight loss endeavors. You can do it! I believe in you.

L.B. Daniels